THIS MIGRAINE TRACKER BELONGS TO

. . . .

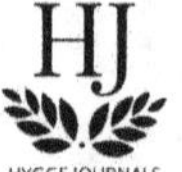
HJ
HYGGE JOURNALS

MIGRAINE symptoms tracker

DATE : **TIME :**

WARNING SIGNS

TYPE OF PAIN

OTHER SYMPTOMS

right   left   left   right

PAIN INTENSITY (FROM LOW TO HIGH) 1 2 3 4 5 6 7 8 9 10

MEDICATIONS & TREATMENT

WHAT WORKED BEST

HOURS OF SLEEP: WEATHER: AIR PRESSURE High / Low

FOOD & BEVERAGE: POSSIBLE TRIGGERS

Other notes and comments:

MIGRAINE symptoms tracker

DATE :   TIME   :

WARNING SIGNS   **TYPE OF PAIN**   **OTHER SYMPTOMS**

right   left   left   right

PAIN INTENSITY (FROM LOW TO HIGH) 1 2 3 4 5 6 7 8 9 10

MEDICATIONS & TREATMENT   **WHAT WORKED BEST**

HOURS OF SLEEP: WEATHER: AIR PRESSURE High / Low

FOOD & BEVERAGE: POSSIBLE TRIGGERS

Other notes and comments:

MIGRAINE symptoms tracker

DATE :   **TIME   :**

WARNING SIGNS   **TYPE OF PAIN**   **OTHER SYMPTOMS**

right   left   left   right

PAIN INTENSITY (FROM LOW TO HIGH) 1 2 3 4 5 6 7 8 9 10

MEDICATIONS & TREATMENT   **WHAT WORKED BEST**

HOURS OF SLEEP: WEATHER: AIR PRESSURE High / Low

FOOD & BEVERAGE: POSSIBLE TRIGGERS

Other notes and comments:

MIGRAINE symptoms tracker

DATE :   TIME   :

WARNING SIGNS	TYPE OF PAIN	OTHER SYMPTOMS

right   left   left   right

PAIN INTENSITY (FROM LOW TO HIGH) 1 2 3 4 5 6 7 8 9 10

MEDICATIONS & TREATMENT   WHAT WORKED BEST

HOURS OF SLEEP: WEATHER: AIR PRESSURE High / Low

FOOD & BEVERAGE: POSSIBLE TRIGGERS

Other notes and comments:

MIGRAINE symptoms tracker

DATE :   **TIME   :**

WARNING SIGNS   **TYPE OF PAIN**   **OTHER SYMPTOMS**

right   left   left   right

PAIN INTENSITY (FROM LOW TO HIGH) 1   2   3   4   5   6   7   8   9   10

MEDICATIONS & TREATMENT   **WHAT WORKED BEST**

HOURS OF SLEEP: WEATHER: AIR PRESSURE High / Low

FOOD & BEVERAGE: POSSIBLE TRIGGERS

Other notes and comments:

MIGRAINE symptoms tracker

DATE :

TIME   :

WARNING SIGNS

TYPE OF PAIN

OTHER SYMPTOMS

right   left   left   right

PAIN INTENSITY (FROM LOW TO HIGH) 1   2   3   4   5   6   7   8   9   10

MEDICATIONS & TREATMENT

WHAT WORKED BEST

HOURS OF SLEEP: WEATHER: AIR PRESSURE High / Low

FOOD & BEVERAGE: POSSIBLE TRIGGERS

Other notes and comments:

MIGRAINE symptoms tracker

DATE :   **TIME   :**

WARNING SIGNS	TYPE OF PAIN	OTHER SYMPTOMS

right   left   left   right

PAIN INTENSITY (FROM LOW TO HIGH)   1   2   3   4   5   6   7   8   9   10

MEDICATIONS & TREATMENT   WHAT WORKED BEST

HOURS OF SLEEP: WEATHER: AIR PRESSURE High / Low

FOOD & BEVERAGE: POSSIBLE TRIGGERS

Other notes and comments:

MIGRAINE symptoms tracker

DATE :

TIME :

WARNING SIGNS	TYPE OF PAIN	OTHER SYMPTOMS

right   left   left   right

PAIN INTENSITY (FROM LOW TO HIGH) 1 2 3 4 5 6 7 8 9 10

MEDICATIONS & TREATMENT

WHAT WORKED BEST

HOURS OF SLEEP: WEATHER: AIR PRESSURE High / Low

FOOD & BEVERAGE: POSSIBLE TRIGGERS

Other notes and comments:

MIGRAINE symptoms tracker

DATE :

TIME   :

WARNING SIGNS

TYPE OF PAIN

OTHER SYMPTOMS

right left

left right

PAIN INTENSITY (FROM LOW TO HIGH) 1 2 3 4 5 6 7 8 9 10

MEDICATIONS & TREATMENT

WHAT WORKED BEST

HOURS OF SLEEP: WEATHER:

AIR PRESSURE High / Low

FOOD & BEVERAGE:

POSSIBLE TRIGGERS

Other notes and comments:

MIGRAINE symptoms tracker

DATE :   **TIME   :**

WARNING SIGNS	TYPE OF PAIN	OTHER SYMPTOMS

right   left   left   right

PAIN INTENSITY (FROM LOW TO HIGH) 1 2 3 4 5 6 7 8 9 10

MEDICATIONS & TREATMENT   WHAT WORKED BEST

HOURS OF SLEEP: WEATHER: AIR PRESSURE High / Low

FOOD & BEVERAGE: POSSIBLE TRIGGERS

Other notes and comments:

MIGRAINE symptoms tracker

DATE :   **TIME   :**

WARNING SIGNS   **TYPE OF PAIN**   **OTHER SYMPTOMS**

right   left   left   right

PAIN INTENSITY (FROM LOW TO HIGH) 1   2   3   4   5   6   7   8   9   10

MEDICATIONS & TREATMENT   **WHAT WORKED BEST**

HOURS OF SLEEP: WEATHER: AIR PRESSURE High / Low

FOOD & BEVERAGE: POSSIBLE TRIGGERS

Other notes and comments:

MIGRAINE symptoms tracker

DATE :

TIME :

WARNING SIGNS

TYPE OF PAIN

OTHER SYMPTOMS

right   left   left   right

PAIN INTENSITY (FROM LOW TO HIGH) 1 2 3 4 5 6 7 8 9 10

MEDICATIONS & TREATMENT

WHAT WORKED BEST

HOURS OF SLEEP: WEATHER: AIR PRESSURE High / Low

FOOD & BEVERAGE:

POSSIBLE TRIGGERS

Other notes and comments:

MIGRAINE symptoms tracker

DATE :   TIME   :

WARNING SIGNS   TYPE OF PAIN   OTHER SYMPTOMS

right   left   left   right

PAIN INTENSITY (FROM LOW TO HIGH)   1   2   3   4   5   6   7   8   9   10

MEDICATIONS & TREATMENT

WHAT WORKED BEST

HOURS OF SLEEP: WEATHER: AIR PRESSURE High / Low

FOOD & BEVERAGE: POSSIBLE TRIGGERS

Other notes and comments:

MIGRAINE symptoms tracker

DATE :   TIME   :

WARNING SIGNS	TYPE OF PAIN	OTHER SYMPTOMS

right   left   left   right

PAIN INTENSITY (FROM LOW TO HIGH) 1 2 3 4 5 6 7 8 9 10

MEDICATIONS & TREATMENT

WHAT WORKED BEST

HOURS OF SLEEP: WEATHER: AIR PRESSURE High / Low

FOOD & BEVERAGE: POSSIBLE TRIGGERS

Other notes and comments:

MIGRAINE symptoms tracker

DATE :   TIME   :

WARNING SIGNS   TYPE OF PAIN   OTHER SYMPTOMS

right   left   left   right

PAIN INTENSITY (FROM LOW TO HIGH) 1 2 3 4 5 6 7 8 9 10

MEDICATIONS & TREATMENT   WHAT WORKED BEST

HOURS OF SLEEP: WEATHER: AIR PRESSURE High / Low

FOOD & BEVERAGE: POSSIBLE TRIGGERS

Other notes and comments:

MIGRAINE symptoms tracker

DATE :   **TIME   :**

WARNING SIGNS	TYPE OF PAIN	OTHER SYMPTOMS

right   left   left   right

PAIN INTENSITY (FROM LOW TO HIGH) 1 2 3 4 5 6 7 8 9 10

MEDICATIONS & TREATMENT   WHAT WORKED BEST

_______________________________   _______________________
_______________________________   _______________________
_______________________________   _______________________
_______________________________   _______________________

HOURS OF SLEEP: WEATHER: AIR PRESSURE High / Low

FOOD & BEVERAGE: POSSIBLE TRIGGERS

____
____
____
____

Other notes and comments:

____
____
____

MIGRAINE symptoms tracker

DATE :   **TIME   :**

WARNING SIGNS   **TYPE OF PAIN**   **OTHER SYMPTOMS**

right   left   left   right

PAIN INTENSITY (FROM LOW TO HIGH) 1   2   3   4   5   6   7   8   9   10

MEDICATIONS & TREATMENT   **WHAT WORKED BEST**

HOURS OF SLEEP: WEATHER: AIR PRESSURE High / Low

FOOD & BEVERAGE: POSSIBLE TRIGGERS

Other notes and comments:

MIGRAINE symptoms tracker

DATE :   TIME   :

WARNING SIGNS	TYPE OF PAIN	OTHER SYMPTOMS

right   left   left   right

PAIN INTENSITY (FROM LOW TO HIGH) 1   2   3   4   5   6   7   8   9   10

MEDICATIONS & TREATMENT   WHAT WORKED BEST

HOURS OF SLEEP: WEATHER: AIR PRESSURE High / Low

FOOD & BEVERAGE: POSSIBLE TRIGGERS

Other notes and comments:

MIGRAINE symptoms tracker

DATE :   **TIME   :**

WARNING SIGNS   **TYPE OF PAIN**   **OTHER SYMPTOMS**

right   left   left   right

PAIN INTENSITY (FROM LOW TO HIGH) 1   2   3   4   5   6   7   8   9   10

MEDICATIONS & TREATMENT   **WHAT WORKED BEST**

HOURS OF SLEEP: WEATHER: AIR PRESSURE High / Low

FOOD & BEVERAGE: POSSIBLE TRIGGERS

Other notes and comments:

DATE :   **TIME   :**

WARNING SIGNS   **TYPE OF PAIN**   **OTHER SYMPTOMS**

right   left   left   right

PAIN INTENSITY (FROM LOW TO HIGH)   1   2   3   4   5   6   7   8   9   10

MEDICATIONS & TREATMENT   **WHAT WORKED BEST**

HOURS OF SLEEP: WEATHER: AIR PRESSURE High / Low

FOOD & BEVERAGE: POSSIBLE TRIGGERS

Other notes and comments:

MIGRAINE symptoms tracker

DATE :   TIME   :

WARNING SIGNS   TYPE OF PAIN   OTHER SYMPTOMS

right   left   left   right

PAIN INTENSITY (FROM LOW TO HIGH) 1   2   3   4   5   6   7   8   9   10

MEDICATIONS & TREATMENT   WHAT WORKED BEST

HOURS OF SLEEP: WEATHER: AIR PRESSURE High / Low

FOOD & BEVERAGE: POSSIBLE TRIGGERS

Other notes and comments:

MIGRAINE symptoms tracker

DATE :

TIME :

WARNING SIGNS	TYPE OF PAIN	OTHER SYMPTOMS

right   left   left   right

PAIN INTENSITY (FROM LOW TO HIGH)   1   2   3   4   5   6   7   8   9   10

MEDICATIONS & TREATMENT

____

____

____

____

WHAT WORKED BEST

____

____

____

____

HOURS OF SLEEP: WEATHER: AIR PRESSURE High / Low

FOOD & BEVERAGE: POSSIBLE TRIGGERS

Other notes and comments:

____

____

____

____

MIGRAINE symptoms tracker

DATE :   **TIME   :**

WARNING SIGNS   **TYPE OF PAIN**   **OTHER SYMPTOMS**

right   left   left   right

PAIN INTENSITY (FROM LOW TO HIGH)   1   2   3   4   5   6   7   8   9   10

MEDICATIONS & TREATMENT   **WHAT WORKED BEST**

HOURS OF SLEEP: WEATHER: AIR PRESSURE High / Low

FOOD & BEVERAGE: POSSIBLE TRIGGERS

Other notes and comments:

MIGRAINE symptoms tracker

DATE :   **TIME   :**

WARNING SIGNS   **TYPE OF PAIN**   **OTHER SYMPTOMS**

right   left   left   right

PAIN INTENSITY (FROM LOW TO HIGH) 1 2 3 4 5 6 7 8 9 10

MEDICATIONS & TREATMENT   **WHAT WORKED BEST**

HOURS OF SLEEP: WEATHER: AIR PRESSURE High / Low

FOOD & BEVERAGE: POSSIBLE TRIGGERS

Other notes and comments:

MIGRAINE symptoms tracker

DATE : **TIME   :**

WARNING SIGNS

TYPE OF PAIN

OTHER SYMPTOMS

right   left   left   right

PAIN INTENSITY (FROM LOW TO HIGH) 1   2   3   4   5   6   7   8   9   10

MEDICATIONS & TREATMENT

WHAT WORKED BEST

HOURS OF SLEEP: WEATHER: AIR PRESSURE High / Low

FOOD & BEVERAGE: POSSIBLE TRIGGERS

Other notes and comments:

MIGRAINE symptoms tracker

DATE :

TIME :

WARNING SIGNS	TYPE OF PAIN	OTHER SYMPTOMS

right   left

left   right

PAIN INTENSITY (FROM LOW TO HIGH) 1 2 3 4 5 6 7 8 9 10

MEDICATIONS & TREATMENT

WHAT WORKED BEST

HOURS OF SLEEP: WEATHER:

AIR PRESSURE High / Low

FOOD & BEVERAGE:

POSSIBLE TRIGGERS

Other notes and comments:

MIGRAINE symptoms tracker

DATE :   **TIME   :**

WARNING SIGNS   **TYPE OF PAIN**   **OTHER SYMPTOMS**

right   left   left   right

PAIN INTENSITY (FROM LOW TO HIGH) 1   2   3   4   5   6   7   8   9   10

MEDICATIONS & TREATMENT   WHAT WORKED BEST

HOURS OF SLEEP: WEATHER: AIR PRESSURE High / Low

FOOD & BEVERAGE: POSSIBLE TRIGGERS

Other notes and comments:

MIGRAINE symptoms tracker

DATE :   **TIME   :**

WARNING SIGNS   TYPE OF PAIN   OTHER SYMPTOMS

right   left   left   right

PAIN INTENSITY (FROM LOW TO HIGH) 1   2   3   4   5   6   7   8   9   10

MEDICATIONS & TREATMENT   WHAT WORKED BEST

HOURS OF SLEEP: WEATHER: AIR PRESSURE High / Low

FOOD & BEVERAGE: POSSIBLE TRIGGERS

Other notes and comments:

MIGRAINE symptoms tracker

DATE :   **TIME   :**

WARNING SIGNS   **TYPE OF PAIN**   **OTHER SYMPTOMS**

right   left   left   right

PAIN INTENSITY (FROM LOW TO HIGH)   1   2   3   4   5   6   7   8   9   10

MEDICATIONS & TREATMENT   **WHAT WORKED BEST**

HOURS OF SLEEP: WEATHER: AIR PRESSURE High / Low

FOOD & BEVERAGE: POSSIBLE TRIGGERS

Other notes and comments:

MIGRAINE symptoms tracker

DATE :   **TIME   :**

WARNING SIGNS	TYPE OF PAIN	OTHER SYMPTOMS

right   left   left   right

PAIN INTENSITY (FROM LOW TO HIGH) 1   2   3   4   5   6   7   8   9   10

MEDICATIONS & TREATMENT

WHAT WORKED BEST

HOURS OF SLEEP: WEATHER:

AIR PRESSURE High / Low

FOOD & BEVERAGE:

POSSIBLE TRIGGERS

Other notes and comments:

MIGRAINE symptoms tracker

DATE :   TIME   :

WARNING SIGNS	TYPE OF PAIN	OTHER SYMPTOMS

right   left   left   right

PAIN INTENSITY (FROM LOW TO HIGH) 1 2 3 4 5 6 7 8 9 10

MEDICATIONS & TREATMENT

WHAT WORKED BEST

HOURS OF SLEEP: WEATHER: AIR PRESSURE High / Low

FOOD & BEVERAGE: POSSIBLE TRIGGERS

Other notes and comments:

MIGRAINE symptoms tracker

DATE : TIME :

WARNING SIGNS	TYPE OF PAIN	OTHER SYMPTOMS

right   left   left   right

PAIN INTENSITY (FROM LOW TO HIGH) 1 2 3 4 5 6 7 8 9 10

MEDICATIONS & TREATMENT

WHAT WORKED BEST

HOURS OF SLEEP: WEATHER: AIR PRESSURE High / Low

FOOD & BEVERAGE: POSSIBLE TRIGGERS

Other notes and comments:

DATE :   TIME   :

WARNING SIGNS   TYPE OF PAIN   OTHER SYMPTOMS

right   left   left   right

PAIN INTENSITY (FROM LOW TO HIGH)   1   2   3   4   5   6   7   8   9   10

MEDICATIONS & TREATMENT   WHAT WORKED BEST

HOURS OF SLEEP: WEATHER: AIR PRESSURE High / Low

FOOD & BEVERAGE: POSSIBLE TRIGGERS

Other notes and comments:

MIGRAINE symptoms tracker

DATE :   TIME   :

WARNING SIGNS	TYPE OF PAIN	OTHER SYMPTOMS

right   left   left   right

PAIN INTENSITY (FROM LOW TO HIGH) 1 2 3 4 5 6 7 8 9 10

MEDICATIONS & TREATMENT   WHAT WORKED BEST

HOURS OF SLEEP: WEATHER: AIR PRESSURE High / Low

FOOD & BEVERAGE: POSSIBLE TRIGGERS

Other notes and comments:

MIGRAINE symptoms tracker

DATE :   **TIME   :**

WARNING SIGNS   **TYPE OF PAIN**   **OTHER SYMPTOMS**

right   left   left   right

PAIN INTENSITY (FROM LOW TO HIGH)   1   2   3   4   5   6   7   8   9   10

MEDICATIONS & TREATMENT   **WHAT WORKED BEST**

HOURS OF SLEEP: WEATHER: AIR PRESSURE High / Low

FOOD & BEVERAGE: POSSIBLE TRIGGERS

Other notes and comments:

MIGRAINE symptoms tracker

DATE :   TIME   :

WARNING SIGNS   **TYPE OF PAIN**   **OTHER SYMPTOMS**

right   left   left   right

PAIN INTENSITY (FROM LOW TO HIGH) 1 2 3 4 5 6 7 8 9 10

MEDICATIONS & TREATMENT   WHAT WORKED BEST

HOURS OF SLEEP: WEATHER: AIR PRESSURE High / Low

FOOD & BEVERAGE: POSSIBLE TRIGGERS

Other notes and comments:

MIGRAINE symptoms tracker

DATE :

TIME   :

WARNING SIGNS

TYPE OF PAIN

OTHER SYMPTOMS

right   left

left   right

PAIN INTENSITY (FROM LOW TO HIGH) 1 2 3 4 5 6 7 8 9 10

MEDICATIONS & TREATMENT

WHAT WORKED BEST

HOURS OF SLEEP: WEATHER:

AIR PRESSURE High / Low

FOOD & BEVERAGE:

POSSIBLE TRIGGERS

Other notes and comments:

MIGRAINE symptoms tracker

DATE :   **TIME   :**

WARNING SIGNS   **TYPE OF PAIN**   **OTHER SYMPTOMS**

right   left   left   right

PAIN INTENSITY (FROM LOW TO HIGH) 1 2 3 4 5 6 7 8 9 10

MEDICATIONS & TREATMENT   **WHAT WORKED BEST**

HOURS OF SLEEP: WEATHER: AIR PRESSURE High / Low

FOOD & BEVERAGE: POSSIBLE TRIGGERS

Other notes and comments:

MIGRAINE symptoms tracker

DATE :   TIME   :

WARNING SIGNS   TYPE OF PAIN   OTHER SYMPTOMS

right   left   left   right

PAIN INTENSITY (FROM LOW TO HIGH)   1   2   3   4   5   6   7   8   9   10

MEDICATIONS & TREATMENT   WHAT WORKED BEST

HOURS OF SLEEP: WEATHER: AIR PRESSURE High / Low

FOOD & BEVERAGE: POSSIBLE TRIGGERS

Other notes and comments:

MIGRAINE symptoms tracker

DATE :   TIME   :

WARNING SIGNS	TYPE OF PAIN	OTHER SYMPTOMS

right   left   left   right

PAIN INTENSITY (FROM LOW TO HIGH) 1 2 3 4 5 6 7 8 9 10

MEDICATIONS & TREATMENT

WHAT WORKED BEST

HOURS OF SLEEP: WEATHER: AIR PRESSURE High / Low

FOOD & BEVERAGE: POSSIBLE TRIGGERS

Other notes and comments:

MIGRAINE symptoms tracker

DATE :   **TIME   :**

WARNING SIGNS   **TYPE OF PAIN**   **OTHER SYMPTOMS**

right   left   left   right

PAIN INTENSITY (FROM LOW TO HIGH) 1   2   3   4   5   6   7   8   9   10

MEDICATIONS & TREATMENT   **WHAT WORKED BEST**

HOURS OF SLEEP: WEATHER: AIR PRESSURE High / Low

FOOD & BEVERAGE: POSSIBLE TRIGGERS

Other notes and comments:

MIGRAINE symptoms tracker

DATE :   TIME   :

WARNING SIGNS	TYPE OF PAIN	OTHER SYMPTOMS

right   left   left   right

PAIN INTENSITY (FROM LOW TO HIGH) 1   2   3   4   5   6   7   8   9   10

MEDICATIONS & TREATMENT

WHAT WORKED BEST

HOURS OF SLEEP: WEATHER:

AIR PRESSURE High / Low

FOOD & BEVERAGE:

POSSIBLE TRIGGERS

Other notes and comments:

MIGRAINE symptoms tracker

DATE :   **TIME   :**

WARNING SIGNS	TYPE OF PAIN	OTHER SYMPTOMS

right   left   left   right

PAIN INTENSITY (FROM LOW TO HIGH) 1 2 3 4 5 6 7 8 9 10

MEDICATIONS & TREATMENT

WHAT WORKED BEST

HOURS OF SLEEP: WEATHER: AIR PRESSURE High / Low

FOOD & BEVERAGE: POSSIBLE TRIGGERS

Other notes and comments:

MIGRAINE symptoms tracker

DATE :   **TIME   :**

WARNING SIGNS   **TYPE OF PAIN**   **OTHER SYMPTOMS**

PAIN INTENSITY (FROM LOW TO HIGH)   1   2   3   4   5   6   7   8   9   10

MEDICATIONS & TREATMENT   WHAT WORKED BEST

HOURS OF SLEEP: WEATHER: AIR PRESSURE High / Low

FOOD & BEVERAGE: POSSIBLE TRIGGERS

Other notes and comments:

MIGRAINE symptoms tracker

DATE :   **TIME   :**

WARNING SIGNS | TYPE OF PAIN | OTHER SYMPTOMS

right   left   left   right

PAIN INTENSITY (FROM LOW TO HIGH) 1   2   3   4   5   6   7   8   9   10

MEDICATIONS & TREATMENT

WHAT WORKED BEST

HOURS OF SLEEP: WEATHER: AIR PRESSURE High / Low

FOOD & BEVERAGE: POSSIBLE TRIGGERS

Other notes and comments:

MIGRAINE symptoms tracker

DATE :   **TIME   :**

WARNING SIGNS   TYPE OF PAIN   OTHER SYMPTOMS

PAIN INTENSITY (FROM LOW TO HIGH) 1 2 3 4 5 6 7 8 9 10

MEDICATIONS & TREATMENT   WHAT WORKED BEST

HOURS OF SLEEP: WEATHER: AIR PRESSURE High / Low

FOOD & BEVERAGE: POSSIBLE TRIGGERS

Other notes and comments:

MIGRAINE symptoms tracker

DATE :   TIME   :

WARNING SIGNS	TYPE OF PAIN	OTHER SYMPTOMS

right   left   left   right

PAIN INTENSITY (FROM LOW TO HIGH)   1   2   3   4   5   6   7   8   9   10

MEDICATIONS & TREATMENT   WHAT WORKED BEST

HOURS OF SLEEP: WEATHER: AIR PRESSURE   High / Low

FOOD & BEVERAGE: POSSIBLE TRIGGERS

Other notes and comments:

MIGRAINE symptoms tracker

DATE :   TIME   :

WARNING SIGNS	TYPE OF PAIN	OTHER SYMPTOMS

right   left   left   right

PAIN INTENSITY (FROM LOW TO HIGH) 1 2 3 4 5 6 7 8 9 10

MEDICATIONS & TREATMENT   WHAT WORKED BEST

HOURS OF SLEEP: WEATHER: AIR PRESSURE High / Low

FOOD & BEVERAGE: POSSIBLE TRIGGERS

Other notes and comments:

MIGRAINE symptoms tracker

DATE :   **TIME   :**

WARNING SIGNS	TYPE OF PAIN	OTHER SYMPTOMS

right   left   left   right

PAIN INTENSITY (FROM LOW TO HIGH) 1   2   3   4   5   6   7   8   9   10

MEDICATIONS & TREATMENT

WHAT WORKED BEST

HOURS OF SLEEP: WEATHER: AIR PRESSURE High / Low

FOOD & BEVERAGE: POSSIBLE TRIGGERS

Other notes and comments:

MIGRAINE symptoms tracker

DATE :   **TIME   :**

WARNING SIGNS   **TYPE OF PAIN**   **OTHER SYMPTOMS**

right   left   left   right

PAIN INTENSITY (FROM LOW TO HIGH) 1 2 3 4 5 6 7 8 9 10

MEDICATIONS & TREATMENT   **WHAT WORKED BEST**

HOURS OF SLEEP: WEATHER: AIR PRESSURE High / Low

FOOD & BEVERAGE: POSSIBLE TRIGGERS

Other notes and comments:

DATE :

TIME   :

WARNING SIGNS

TYPE OF PAIN

OTHER SYMPTOMS

PAIN INTENSITY (FROM LOW TO HIGH)   1   2   3   4   5   6   7   8   9   10

MEDICATIONS & TREATMENT

WHAT WORKED BEST

HOURS OF SLEEP: WEATHER:

AIR PRESSURE High / Low

FOOD & BEVERAGE:

POSSIBLE TRIGGERS

Other notes and comments:

MIGRAINE symptoms tracker

DATE :   **TIME   :**

WARNING SIGNS   **TYPE OF PAIN**   **OTHER SYMPTOMS**

right   left   left   right

PAIN INTENSITY (FROM LOW TO HIGH) 1 2 3 4 5 6 7 8 9 10

MEDICATIONS & TREATMENT   WHAT WORKED BEST

HOURS OF SLEEP: WEATHER: AIR PRESSURE High / Low

FOOD & BEVERAGE: POSSIBLE TRIGGERS

Other notes and comments:

MIGRAINE symptoms tracker

DATE :

TIME   :

WARNING SIGNS	TYPE OF PAIN	OTHER SYMPTOMS

right   left   left   right

PAIN INTENSITY (FROM LOW TO HIGH)   1   2   3   4   5   6   7   8   9   10

MEDICATIONS & TREATMENT

WHAT WORKED BEST

HOURS OF SLEEP: WEATHER: AIR PRESSURE High / Low

FOOD & BEVERAGE: POSSIBLE TRIGGERS

Other notes and comments:

MIGRAINE symptoms tracker

DATE :   **TIME   :**

WARNING SIGNS	TYPE OF PAIN	OTHER SYMPTOMS

right   left   left   right

PAIN INTENSITY (FROM LOW TO HIGH)   1   2   3   4   5   6   7   8   9   10

MEDICATIONS & TREATMENT   **WHAT WORKED BEST**

HOURS OF SLEEP: WEATHER: AIR PRESSURE High / Low

FOOD & BEVERAGE: POSSIBLE TRIGGERS

Other notes and comments:

MIGRAINE symptoms tracker

DATE :   TIME   :

WARNING SIGNS   TYPE OF PAIN   OTHER SYMPTOMS

right   left   left   right

PAIN INTENSITY (FROM LOW TO HIGH) 1 2 3 4 5 6 7 8 9 10

MEDICATIONS & TREATMENT   WHAT WORKED BEST

HOURS OF SLEEP: WEATHER: AIR PRESSURE High / Low

FOOD & BEVERAGE: POSSIBLE TRIGGERS

Other notes and comments:

MIGRAINE symptoms tracker

DATE :   TIME   :

WARNING SIGNS	TYPE OF PAIN	OTHER SYMPTOMS

right   left   left   right

PAIN INTENSITY (FROM LOW TO HIGH) 1 2 3 4 5 6 7 8 9 10

MEDICATIONS & TREATMENT   WHAT WORKED BEST

HOURS OF SLEEP: WEATHER: AIR PRESSURE High / Low

FOOD & BEVERAGE: POSSIBLE TRIGGERS

Other notes and comments:

MIGRAINE symptoms tracker

DATE : **TIME :**

WARNING SIGNS

TYPE OF PAIN

OTHER SYMPTOMS

right left left right

PAIN INTENSITY (FROM LOW TO HIGH) 1 2 3 4 5 6 7 8 9 10

MEDICATIONS & TREATMENT

WHAT WORKED BEST

HOURS OF SLEEP: WEATHER: AIR PRESSURE High / Low

FOOD & BEVERAGE: POSSIBLE TRIGGERS

Other notes and comments:

MIGRAINE symptoms tracker

DATE :   TIME   :

WARNING SIGNS	TYPE OF PAIN	OTHER SYMPTOMS

right   left   left   right

PAIN INTENSITY (FROM LOW TO HIGH) 1 2 3 4 5 6 7 8 9 10

MEDICATIONS & TREATMENT   WHAT WORKED BEST

HOURS OF SLEEP: WEATHER: AIR PRESSURE High / Low

FOOD & BEVERAGE: POSSIBLE TRIGGERS

Other notes and comments:

MIGRAINE symptoms tracker

DATE :   TIME   :

WARNING SIGNS	TYPE OF PAIN	OTHER SYMPTOMS

right   left   left   right

PAIN INTENSITY (FROM LOW TO HIGH)   1   2   3   4   5   6   7   8   9   10

MEDICATIONS & TREATMENT

WHAT WORKED BEST

HOURS OF SLEEP: WEATHER: AIR PRESSURE High / Low

FOOD & BEVERAGE: POSSIBLE TRIGGERS

Other notes and comments:

MIGRAINE symptoms tracker

DATE :   TIME   :

WARNING SIGNS	TYPE OF PAIN	OTHER SYMPTOMS

right   left   left   right

PAIN INTENSITY (FROM LOW TO HIGH) 1   2   3   4   5   6   7   8   9   10

MEDICATIONS & TREATMENT   WHAT WORKED BEST

HOURS OF SLEEP: WEATHER: AIR PRESSURE High / Low

FOOD & BEVERAGE: POSSIBLE TRIGGERS

Other notes and comments:

MIGRAINE symptoms tracker

DATE :   TIME   :

WARNING SIGNS	TYPE OF PAIN	OTHER SYMPTOMS

right   left   left   right

PAIN INTENSITY (FROM LOW TO HIGH) 1 2 3 4 5 6 7 8 9 10

MEDICATIONS & TREATMENT

WHAT WORKED BEST

HOURS OF SLEEP: WEATHER: AIR PRESSURE High / Low

FOOD & BEVERAGE: POSSIBLE TRIGGERS

Other notes and comments:

MIGRAINE symptoms tracker

DATE :   **TIME   :**

WARNING SIGNS	TYPE OF PAIN	OTHER SYMPTOMS

right   left   left   right

PAIN INTENSITY (FROM LOW TO HIGH) 1   2   3   4   5   6   7   8   9   10

MEDICATIONS & TREATMENT   **WHAT WORKED BEST**

HOURS OF SLEEP: WEATHER: AIR PRESSURE High / Low

FOOD & BEVERAGE: POSSIBLE TRIGGERS

Other notes and comments:

MIGRAINE symptoms tracker

DATE :   TIME   :

WARNING SIGNS   TYPE OF PAIN   OTHER SYMPTOMS

PAIN INTENSITY (FROM LOW TO HIGH) 1 2 3 4 5 6 7 8 9 10

MEDICATIONS & TREATMENT   WHAT WORKED BEST

HOURS OF SLEEP: WEATHER: AIR PRESSURE High / Low

FOOD & BEVERAGE: POSSIBLE TRIGGERS

Other notes and comments:

DATE :   TIME   :

WARNING SIGNS   TYPE OF PAIN   OTHER SYMPTOMS

right   left   left   right

PAIN INTENSITY (FROM LOW TO HIGH) 1   2   3   4   5   6   7   8   9   10

MEDICATIONS & TREATMENT   WHAT WORKED BEST

HOURS OF SLEEP: WEATHER: AIR PRESSURE High / Low

FOOD & BEVERAGE: POSSIBLE TRIGGERS

Other notes and comments:

MIGRAINE symptoms tracker

DATE :   TIME   :

WARNING SIGNS	TYPE OF PAIN	OTHER SYMPTOMS

right   left   left   right

PAIN INTENSITY (FROM LOW TO HIGH) 1   2   3   4   5   6   7   8   9   10

MEDICATIONS & TREATMENT

WHAT WORKED BEST

HOURS OF SLEEP: WEATHER: AIR PRESSURE High / Low

FOOD & BEVERAGE: POSSIBLE TRIGGERS

Other notes and comments:

MIGRAINE symptoms tracker

DATE :   **TIME   :**

WARNING SIGNS	TYPE OF PAIN	OTHER SYMPTOMS

right   left   left   right

PAIN INTENSITY (FROM LOW TO HIGH) 1 2 3 4 5 6 7 8 9 10

MEDICATIONS & TREATMENT   WHAT WORKED BEST

HOURS OF SLEEP: WEATHER: AIR PRESSURE High / Low

FOOD & BEVERAGE: POSSIBLE TRIGGERS

Other notes and comments:

MIGRAINE symptoms tracker

DATE :   **TIME   :**

WARNING SIGNS   **TYPE OF PAIN**   **OTHER SYMPTOMS**

right   left   left   right

PAIN INTENSITY (FROM LOW TO HIGH) 1   2   3   4   5   6   7   8   9   10

MEDICATIONS & TREATMENT   **WHAT WORKED BEST**

HOURS OF SLEEP: WEATHER: AIR PRESSURE High / Low

FOOD & BEVERAGE: POSSIBLE TRIGGERS

Other notes and comments:

MIGRAINE symptoms tracker

DATE :   TIME   :

WARNING SIGNS	TYPE OF PAIN	OTHER SYMPTOMS

right   left   left   right

PAIN INTENSITY (FROM LOW TO HIGH) 1 2 3 4 5 6 7 8 9 10

MEDICATIONS & TREATMENT   WHAT WORKED BEST

HOURS OF SLEEP: WEATHER: AIR PRESSURE High / Low

FOOD & BEVERAGE: POSSIBLE TRIGGERS

Other notes and comments:

MIGRAINE symptoms tracker

DATE :   TIME   :

WARNING SIGNS	TYPE OF PAIN	OTHER SYMPTOMS

right   left   left   right

PAIN INTENSITY (FROM LOW TO HIGH) 1 2 3 4 5 6 7 8 9 10

MEDICATIONS & TREATMENT

WHAT WORKED BEST

HOURS OF SLEEP: WEATHER: AIR PRESSURE High / Low

FOOD & BEVERAGE: POSSIBLE TRIGGERS

Other notes and comments:

DATE :

TIME   :

WARNING SIGNS

TYPE OF PAIN

OTHER SYMPTOMS

right   left   left   right

PAIN INTENSITY (FROM LOW TO HIGH) 1 2 3 4 5 6 7 8 9 10

MEDICATIONS & TREATMENT

WHAT WORKED BEST

HOURS OF SLEEP: WEATHER: AIR PRESSURE High / Low

FOOD & BEVERAGE: POSSIBLE TRIGGERS

Other notes and comments:

MIGRAINE symptoms tracker

DATE :   **TIME   :**

WARNING SIGNS	TYPE OF PAIN	OTHER SYMPTOMS

right   left   left   right

PAIN INTENSITY (FROM LOW TO HIGH) 1 2 3 4 5 6 7 8 9 10

MEDICATIONS & TREATMENT   WHAT WORKED BEST

HOURS OF SLEEP: WEATHER: AIR PRESSURE High / Low

FOOD & BEVERAGE: POSSIBLE TRIGGERS

Other notes and comments:

MIGRAINE symptoms tracker

DATE :   TIME   :

WARNING SIGNS	TYPE OF PAIN	OTHER SYMPTOMS

right   left   left   right

PAIN INTENSITY (FROM LOW TO HIGH) 1 2 3 4 5 6 7 8 9 10

MEDICATIONS & TREATMENT   WHAT WORKED BEST

HOURS OF SLEEP: WEATHER: AIR PRESSURE High / Low

FOOD & BEVERAGE: POSSIBLE TRIGGERS

Other notes and comments:

MIGRAINE symptoms tracker

DATE :   TIME   :

WARNING SIGNS   TYPE OF PAIN   OTHER SYMPTOMS

right   left   left   right

PAIN INTENSITY (FROM LOW TO HIGH)   1   2   3   4   5   6   7   8   9   10

MEDICATIONS & TREATMENT   WHAT WORKED BEST

HOURS OF SLEEP: WEATHER: AIR PRESSURE High / Low

FOOD & BEVERAGE: POSSIBLE TRIGGERS

Other notes and comments:

MIGRAINE symptoms tracker

DATE :   TIME   :

WARNING SIGNS   TYPE OF PAIN   OTHER SYMPTOMS

PAIN INTENSITY (FROM LOW TO HIGH) 1 2 3 4 5 6 7 8 9 10

MEDICATIONS & TREATMENT   WHAT WORKED BEST

HOURS OF SLEEP: WEATHER: AIR PRESSURE High / Low

FOOD & BEVERAGE: POSSIBLE TRIGGERS

Other notes and comments:

MIGRAINE symptoms tracker

DATE :   **TIME   :**

WARNING SIGNS   **TYPE OF PAIN**   **OTHER SYMPTOMS**

right   left   left   right

PAIN INTENSITY (FROM LOW TO HIGH) 1   2   3   4   5   6   7   8   9   10

MEDICATIONS & TREATMENT   **WHAT WORKED BEST**

HOURS OF SLEEP: WEATHER: AIR PRESSURE High / Low

FOOD & BEVERAGE: POSSIBLE TRIGGERS

Other notes and comments:

MIGRAINE symptoms tracker

DATE :   TIME   :

| WARNING SIGNS | TYPE OF PAIN | OTHER SYMPTOMS |

right   left   left   right

PAIN INTENSITY (FROM LOW TO HIGH)   1   2   3   4   5   6   7   8   9   10

MEDICATIONS & TREATMENT   WHAT WORKED BEST

HOURS OF SLEEP: WEATHER: AIR PRESSURE High / Low

FOOD & BEVERAGE: POSSIBLE TRIGGERS

Other notes and comments:

MIGRAINE symptoms tracker

DATE :   **TIME   :**

WARNING SIGNS   **TYPE OF PAIN**   **OTHER SYMPTOMS**

right   left   left   right

PAIN INTENSITY (FROM LOW TO HIGH)   1   2   3   4   5   6   7   8   9   10

MEDICATIONS & TREATMENT   **WHAT WORKED BEST**

HOURS OF SLEEP: WEATHER: AIR PRESSURE High / Low

FOOD & BEVERAGE: POSSIBLE TRIGGERS

Other notes and comments:

MIGRAINE symptoms tracker

DATE :   TIME   :

WARNING SIGNS	TYPE OF PAIN	OTHER SYMPTOMS

right   left   left   right

PAIN INTENSITY (FROM LOW TO HIGH) 1   2   3   4   5   6   7   8   9   10

MEDICATIONS & TREATMENT   WHAT WORKED BEST

HOURS OF SLEEP: WEATHER: AIR PRESSURE High / Low

FOOD & BEVERAGE: POSSIBLE TRIGGERS

Other notes and comments:

DATE :

TIME   :

WARNING SIGNS

TYPE OF PAIN

OTHER SYMPTOMS

right   left   left   right

PAIN INTENSITY (FROM LOW TO HIGH)   1   2   3   4   5   6   7   8   9   10

MEDICATIONS & TREATMENT

WHAT WORKED BEST

HOURS OF SLEEP: WEATHER: AIR PRESSURE High / Low

FOOD & BEVERAGE:

POSSIBLE TRIGGERS

Other notes and comments:

MIGRAINE symptoms tracker

DATE :   TIME   :

WARNING SIGNS	TYPE OF PAIN	OTHER SYMPTOMS

right   left   left   right

PAIN INTENSITY (FROM LOW TO HIGH) 1 2 3 4 5 6 7 8 9 10

MEDICATIONS & TREATMENT   WHAT WORKED BEST

HOURS OF SLEEP: WEATHER: AIR PRESSURE High / Low

FOOD & BEVERAGE: POSSIBLE TRIGGERS

Other notes and comments:

MIGRAINE symptoms tracker

DATE :   TIME   :

WARNING SIGNS   TYPE OF PAIN   OTHER SYMPTOMS

right   left   left   right

PAIN INTENSITY (FROM LOW TO HIGH)   1   2   3   4   5   6   7   8   9   10

MEDICATIONS & TREATMENT   WHAT WORKED BEST

HOURS OF SLEEP: WEATHER: AIR PRESSURE High / Low

FOOD & BEVERAGE: POSSIBLE TRIGGERS

Other notes and comments:

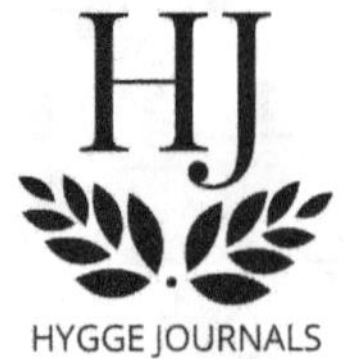

HJ
HYGGE JOURNALS